Smallpox and the American Indian

by
Arthur Diamond

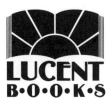

LUCENT
B·O·O·K·S

These and other titles are available in the Lucent World Disaster Series:

The Armenian Earthquake	**The Exxon-Valdez Oil Spill**
The Bhopal Chemical Leak	**The Hindenburg**
The Black Death	**Hiroshima**
The Challenger	**The Irish Potato Famine**
Chernobyl	**Krakatoa**
The Chicago Fire	**The Lockerbie Airline Crash**
The Children's Crusade	**Pompeii**
The Crash of 1929	**The San Francisco Earthquake**
The Dust Bowl	**Smallpox and the American Indian**
The Ethiopian Famine	**The Titanic**

Acknowledgement
The author thanks Kate Guzman for friendship and inspiration.

Library of Congress Cataloging-in-Publication Data

Diamond, Arthur, 1957-
    Smallpox and the American Indian / by Arthur Diamond.
      p. cm. — (World disasters)
    Includes bibliographical references and index.
    Summary: Describes the series of smallpox epidemics that
decimated Native American populations in the 1800's.
    ISBN 1-56006-018-2
    1. Indians of North America—West (U.S.)—Diseases—Social
aspects—Juvenile literature. 2. Indians of North America—West
(U.S.)—Population—Juvenile literature. 3. Smallpox—West
(U.S.)—Juvenile literature. I. Title. II. Series.
E98.D6D53   1991
978'.00497—dc20   91-23066
                                                                CIP
                                                                 AC

To my dear friends Gary, Shannon, Erin, and Lissa Rubin

Table of Contents

Preface
The World Disasters Series

World disasters have always aroused human curiosity. Whenever news of tragedy spreads, we want to learn more about it. We wonder how and why the disaster happened, how people reacted, and whether we might have acted differently. To be sure, disaster evokes a wide range of responses—fear, sorrow, despair, generosity, even hope. Yet from every great disaster, one remarkable truth always seems to emerge: in spite of death, pain, and destruction, the human spirit triumphs.

History is full of disasters, arising from a variety of causes. Earthquakes, floods, volcanic eruptions, and other natural events often produce widespread destruction. Just as often, however, people accidentally bring suffering and distress on themselves and other human beings. And many disasters have sinister causes, like human greed, envy, or prejudice.

The disasters included in this series have been chosen not only for their dramatic qualities, but also for their educational value. The reader will learn about the causes and effects of the greatest disasters in history. Technical concepts and interesting anecdotes are explained and illustrated in inset boxes.

But disasters should not be viewed in isolation. To enrich the reader's understanding, these books present historical information about the time period, and interesting facts about the culture in which each disaster occurred. Finally, they teach valuable lessons about human nature. More acts of bravery, cowardice, intelligence, and foolishness are compressed into the few days of a disaster than most people experience in a lifetime.

Dramatic illustrations and evocative narrative lure the reader to distant cities and times gone by. Readers witness the awesome power of an exploding volcano, the magnitude of a violent earthquake, and the hopelessness of passengers on a mighty ship passing to its watery grave. By reliving the events, the reader will see how disaster affects the lives of real people and will gain a deeper understanding of their sorrow, their pain, their courage, and their hope.

Introduction

Silence over the Prairie

By the time Columbus began his travels toward North America, Native Americans had inhabited every livable region of that continent for many centuries. More than three hundred years later, in 1836, white settlers occupied some of the land, but the wilderness still belonged to the Indians, from Alaska down to Mexico, from the Missouri River to the great Pacific Ocean.

Contact between whites and Indians began with trade. In the early 1800s, the American Fur Company established trading posts, called forts, along the banks of the Mississippi and Missouri rivers to exchange goods with the Indians. Whites wanted the furs of bears, beavers, and buffalo. The Indians knew how to obtain these furs and traded for blankets, weapons, and other goods.

In the summer of 1837, a steamboat from Saint Louis headed up the Missouri River, carrying goods for trade with the Indians. Members of the Mandan, Assiniboin, and Blackfoot tribes arrived at various forts along the Missouri in anticipation of the boat's arrival. But the Indians did not know that the goods they would receive—copper utensils, flints, tobacco, and alcohol—would be tainted by an invisible killer.

Although the Indians of North America had long suffered from smallpox, the epidemic that lasted from 1837 to 1840 was, as one historian wrote, "possibly the most widespread and devastating of any which have occurred either before or since." It is estimated that from 100,000 to 300,000 Indians died in this plague.

The human suffering was enormous. Whole tribes were wiped out. Family lineages were destroyed. The prairie, once populated with Indians, was deserted except for the wolves and other predators who fed on the uncounted human corpses.

Although this book tells how the epidemic affected the tribes of the upper Missouri River, it destroyed other tribes as well. The tragedy of the Mandan, Assiniboin, and Blackfoot is also the tragedy of the tribes located in Alaska, the Northwest, California, and the Southwest. Why did so many Indians die? Why were there no attempts to stop the plague from spreading? In the end, a combination of factors, including greed, heartlessness, and misunderstanding, led to the downfall of so many Indian cultures.

Smallpox and the American Indian in History

10,000 B.C.
Indian hunting/gathering cultures thrive in North America

1132 B.C.
Egyptian Pharaoh Ramses V dies of smallpox

396 B.C.
Carthaginian army led by Hannibal against Romans is ravaged by epidemic of disease now thought to be smallpox

300 B.C.
Chinese use inoculation to prevent smallpox

A.D. 476
Fall of the Roman Empire

1000
Norwegian explorer Leif Eriksson sails to North America

1096-1219
Crusades

1334
Bubonic plague (Black Death) begins in Europe and Asia

1492
Christopher Columbus arrives in the New World

1607
John Smith establishes first permanent English settlement in North America at Jamestown, Virginia

1621
Pilgrims celebrate first Thanksgiving with Indians at Plymouth, Massachusetts

1626
Carnarsee Indians sell Manhattan Island, which belongs to Manhattan Indians, to white settlers for about $24 worth of goods

1689
King William's War, first in a series of wars waged in North America between England and France. Both nations recruited Indians in the fight

1763
Treaty of Paris ends French and Indian Wars

1776
United States declares independence from Great Britain

1787
Congress passes Northwest Ordinance, making illegal the taking of Indian land and property, except through formal treaty

1797
Edward Jenner develops smallpox vaccine in England

1803
U.S. purchases Louisiana territory from French

1809
Treaty of Fort Wayne cedes 1.5 million acres of Indian land in Indiana and Ohio to U.S. government

1813
Shawnee chief Tecumseh dies fighting for British in War of 1812

1821
Tarborough Affair prevents use of smallpox vaccine in United States

1824
U.S. government establishes Bureau of Indian Affairs to ensure fair treatment of Indians by whites

1830
Andrew Jackson enacts Indian Removal Act to move Indians out of territories settled by whites

1837
Trading ship *St. Peter* brings smallpox to Plains Indians, setting off four-year epidemic decimating Indian populations

1838
During smallpox epidemic, Massachusetts repeals quarantine law requiring isolation of persons with smallpox

1848
U.S. acquires California, Arizona, New Mexico, Utah, Nevada, and Texas in Mexican-American War

1861
U.S. Civil War begins

1866
Railroad Enabling Act allows railroads to take Indian land for railroad construction

1867
Russia sells Alaska to the U.S.

1876
Sioux defeat Custer's troops in Battle of the Little Bighorn

1890
U.S. Army massacres 300 Sioux at Wounded Knee, South Dakota

1914
World War I begins

1924
Congress makes Native Americans full citizens; they are given the right to vote in local, state, and federal elections

1934
Congress passes Indian Reorganization Act. The act recognizes Native Americans' right to self-determination, allows them to purchase land and makes the selling of tribal lands dependent on tribal, not individual, agreement

1939
World War II begins

1979
World Health Organization announces smallpox totally eradicated

1980
U.S. Indian population measured at 1,534,000

1987
Federal government lists 861,500 Indians living on reservations

1990
Native American Graves and Repatriation Act passed. Act allows Native Americans to retrieve tribal objects from museums

1991
Movie *Dances with Wolves* engages millions of Americans in the historical plight of the Indians' treatment by U.S. government

One

Indian Country

The first half of the nineteenth century was one of rapid growth and westward expansion in the United States. As population increased and immigrants continued to arrive from Europe, the federal government encouraged the development of the frontier.

In 1803, the U.S. acquired the Louisiana Territory from France, which opened up the way for expansion to the West. Occupying about the entire middle third of the present-day continental United States, this huge area of more than 827,000 square miles of land doubled the size of the country. Seeking information about the new territory and the area beyond, in 1804, President Thomas Jefferson sent explorers Meriwether Lewis and William Clark on an expedition from Saint Louis to the Pacific coast. The expedition discovered, met, and traded with various Indian tribes along the way. This opened the way for future trade between the Indians and the traders and trappers who would follow.

Exploration Encouraged

The federal government continued to encourage the exploration of the frontier. With government support, the Missouri and Arkansas regions were explored by Henry Schoolcraft in 1818 and 1819. In 1818 and 1819, Maj. Stephen Long set out to map the Great Plains, and beginning in 1827, railroad routes were mapped out through the wilderness.

To promote settlement in the new areas, the government priced land at two dollars an acre—a relatively high price—but offered a payment plan that made it affordable.

All across the country, Americans steadily advanced into the frontier. In Florida, white settlers edged into the swamps of the Everglades. In 1848, Mexico ceded California to the United States, and American settlements were established. Even in Russian Alaska, American settlers and traders pushed into the wilderness.

In the 1830s, in the eastern part of North America, a network of inland waterways aided the settlement of the country's vast interior. Steamboats were able to maneuver slowly up the Missouri River and carry goods far into the country, from cities such as Saint Louis.

In the 1830s, the Missouri River,

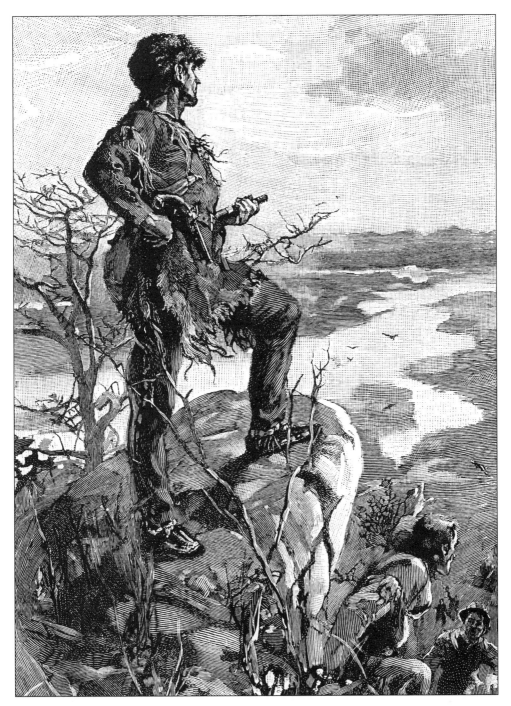

Meriwether Lewis gazes out over the Rocky Mountains. At the request of President Thomas Jefferson, Lewis and William Clark led an expedition to explore the western frontier in 1804.

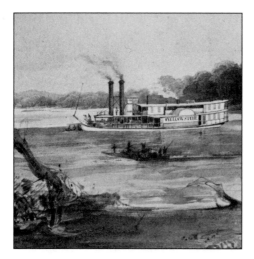

Before the railroad, steamboats provided an essential form of transportation. Steamboats traveled the Mississippi, Missouri, and other main waterways.

or "Big Muddy," was a magnificent waterway. Going up the river, travelers witnessed beautiful and clean rushing springs, pine trees smelling sweet in the sun, and exquisite secret meadows alive with wildflowers. The forests rustled with the activities of bears and beavers, and the prairies echoed with the thunder of hooves from the huge herds of antelope, deer, and buffalo. From Saint Louis, steamboats traveled the river northwest through wilderness now known as Nebraska, South Dakota, North Dakota, and Montana.

The American Fur Company, founded by John Jacob Astor, built many trading posts along the Missouri River. Agents of the company transported guns and ammunition, tobacco, red beads, and cloth from Saint Louis on a regular basis to trade for the elk skins, beaver and muskrat pelts, dried buffalo meat, and buffalo robes that the Indians brought to the posts.

The Indians

In 1836, 4.5 million Indians lived in North America. They were divided into tribes that were further divided into bands. Indian territory was divided into six broad areas: Eastern Woodlands, Southwest, Plateau, Northwest Coast, North or Subarctic, and the Plains.

The vast Plains area spread from the Mississippi River to the Rocky Mountains. It was a land of wide prairies grazed by huge herds of buffalo. Fertile grasslands stretched farther than the eye could see. Summers were warm on the plains, and the winters bitterly cold.

Several nomadic, or wandering, Plains Indian tribes, including the Sioux, Assiniboin, Blackfoot, and Gros Ventres, came seasonally to the forts on the banks of the Missouri River to trade with the whites. Other Plains Indian tribes, like the Arikara and the Hidatsa, had permanent settlements on the river. One of the largest tribes with permanent settlements along the banks of the Missouri was the Mandan.

The Mandan

The Mandan lived in two villages, one slightly larger than the other, on the forested banks of the Missouri River, just below the mouth of the Big Knife River, in what is modern-day North Dakota. In order to survive, they ventured out on the prairie to hunt buffalo, but mostly they ate what they could grow near

THE BUFFALO

Indians depended on their environment to provide their food, shelter, and clothing. A river valley, with its supply of water and fertile soil, was an ideal environment for farming. The plains, however, were a more hostile environment, without abundant water supplies, fertile soil, or usable timber. The source of life for the Blackfoot and other Plains Indian tribes was the buffalo.

Every part of the buffalo was used in daily life. Hides were tanned and made into tepees, clothing, and blankets; hair was used for weaving; horns and bones were carved into weapons and utensils; and the belly was turned into a giant cooking pot. Buffalo meat was the staple of the Blackfoot diet.

The buffalo hunt was a ritual for the Blackfoot. First, a buffalo dance would be performed. Wearing war paint, members of the tribe would put on the skins of buffalo and imitate their movements in a ritual dance. This was believed to lure the animals to the tribe's hunting grounds.

On a buffalo hunt, large parties of Blackfoot would venture out on the prairie on horseback, looking for a large herd. They would usually not go more than forty miles or so from their village for fear of attack by other tribes.

After spotting a large herd of buffalo, the Blackfoot usually attacked on horseback, shooting arrows. Other methods were also tried, such as dressing in wolf skins and creeping as close to the herds as possible before attacking. Also, a herd could be driven over a cliff or into an enclosure, where it would be surrounded and slaughtered. The meat was stripped at the scene of the hunt and usually dried there, then taken back to the village.

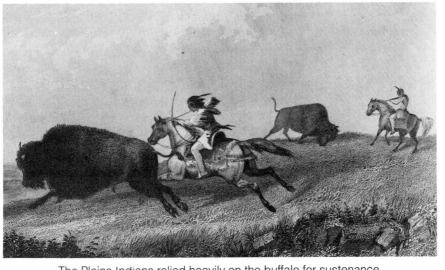

The Plains Indians relied heavily on the buffalo for sustenance.

the river—maize, squash, beans, and sunflowers.

The Mandan were described by those whites who saw them as taller than other Indians, with light skin. Their noses were said to be shorter than those of the Sioux and not as arched, and their cheekbones were lower. They had dark, narrow eyes. Men and women wore robes and

11

aprons of buffalo skin as well as deerskin leggings and moccasins. Both sexes paid special attention to their hair, which they ornamented with braids and feathers.

Earth Lodges

The Mandan lived in earth lodges, which were square structures made of crossed poles and hay and covered with hard, waterproof clay. Lodges could be from thirty to sixty feet in diameter, and each had a smoke hole in the roof. Each village contained from thirty to seventy lodges, grouped closely together and facing a large plaza.

Also on the edge of the plaza were ceremonial lodges, with a ceremonial post out in front where ritual dancing would take place. The Mandan used ritual dancing to communicate with their gods and ask for success in hunting or victory in war.

The Mandan villages were in the midst of Sioux country. The Mandan had no doubt, however, that the land was their rightful home. According to tribal legend, the Mandan were led from underground to the surface by a being named Good Furred Robe and his brothers and sisters.

Because they lived so close to one another, tribes of the upper Missouri were almost always at war. The Sioux would attack the Mandan and their neighbors, the Hidatsa and Arikara. Then the Sioux themselves would be attacked, and then a truce would be declared. The truce would be celebrated by a big feast and dancing among the tribes. Soon, though, the tribes would again be at war.

War was popular among the Plains Indians and provided a way for a young brave to rise in the ranks of his tribe. Among the Plains Indians, a warrior had to perform certain acts to become a chief: he must strike an enemy; he must lead a successful raid; he must capture a horse tethered in an enemy camp; and he must take the bow or knife from an enemy in hand-to-hand combat.

Chief Ma-to-toh-pah

Ma-to-toh-pah (Four Bears) was the chief of the Mandan and one of their greatest warriors. He was also a friend of the white settlers, and traders admired him and had no fear of attack from his people.

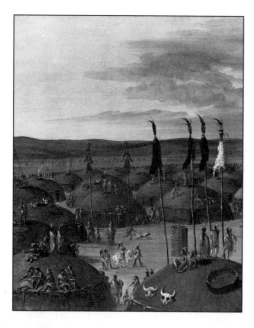

Western artist George Catlin sketched this typical Mandan village in 1837.

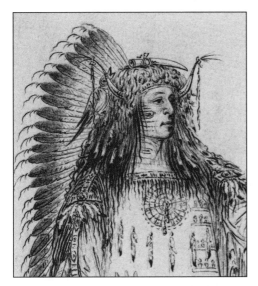

Ma-to-toh-pah became chief of the Mandan tribe in part because of his daring bravery in war.

One observer described Ma-to-toh-pah as "free, generous, elegant and gentlemanly in his deportment—the most extraordinary man, perhaps, who lives at this day, in the atmosphere of Nature's nobleman." One of his admirers was the Western artist George Catlin, who visited and painted portraits of the Mandan leader.

Ma-to-toh-pah's actions in war had elevated him to chief. In one of his more well known exploits, he crept into an Arikara village at night and murdered his brother's killer. He had waited in vain for four years for the chance to meet the killer in battle.

The chiefs of the Plains Indian tribes had scenes of their great deeds woven into the robes they wore, and among the scenes woven into Ma-to-toh-pah's robe was the depiction of a battle with the Cheyenne. After a Cheyenne raid, Ma-to-toh-pah single-handedly challenged the whole Cheyenne war party to battle, even though his tribe was outnumbered. Impressed by this boldness, the Cheyenne chief agreed to fight Ma-to-toh-pah one-on-one, on the condition that each one strip himself of his corresponding weapons before the fight. When they reached their knives, Ma-to-toh-poh was defenseless—he had left his knife back in the village. He grappled with the other man and was able to grab the knife and plunge it into the chest of the stunned Cheyenne leader. This victory was among the many great deeds that made Ma-to-toh-pah a feared and respected figure among neighboring tribes. The traders at nearby Fort Clark also admired and respected the chief.

Fort Clark

Fort Clark was one of the first trading posts established on the upper Missouri River. These outposts for trade were scattered along the great river. Until the mid-1800s, these forts were for trading only and did not serve any military purpose. Under the leadership of Commander F.A. Chardon, Fort Clark was the main Mandan trading post. It was built on the west bank of the Missouri River about eight miles below the mouth of Big Knife River, sixty miles north of modern-day Bismarck, North Dakota. Small, shoddy, and ramshackle, it was located just across the river from the

SQUAWS

The Assiniboin squaw had a life similar to that of squaws in other Plains Indian tribes. Hers was a domestic life: She mostly gathered and prepared food and took care of the children. While it was the brave's role to train and breed horses, the squaw actually owned the herds. Some squaws proved to be great hunters and would compete with the men of their tribe.

Sometimes a squaw would rise to a position of power from within the male-dominated tribes. One such woman, named Woman Chief, lived near the Assiniboin, and, as the historian Elinor Wilson recalls, could "rival any of the young men in all their amusements and occupations, was a capital shot with the rifle, and would spend most of her time in killing deer and bighorn, which she carried home on her back when hunting on foot."

A squaw usually shared her husband with other wives, since the mortality rate among men was high, due to the dangers of continual raids and wars. Some squaws became the wives of traders at forts on the upper Missouri.

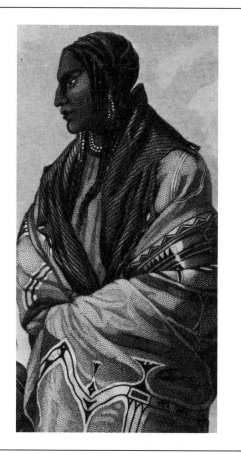

Mandan villages.

Living quarters for resident traders in the fort were made of logs crudely put together. Adjoining sections were built surrounding a central storehouse that was fortified with thick log walls. Traders could retreat to this storehouse if attacked by Indians.

In 1836, Fort Clark also served part of the Assiniboin tribe. The Assiniboin were the northern neighbors of the Mandan. An incident in 1836 cemented a friendship between the two tribes. An Assiniboin trading party, encountering hostile Mandan villagers, was protected from a hail of arrows and gunfire by Chief Ma-to-toh-pah himself.

The Assiniboin ranged in a circular area encompassing Saskatchewan and Winnipeg in Canada and the areas south of the Missouri River. Unlike the Mandan, the Assiniboin were nomads and lived in tepees on the prairie. The tepees were made of buffalo hides sewn together and stretched around poles standing upright in a circle. The Assiniboin camps could be taken down and put back up easily, and the tribe moved often, under the instructions of its leader, Chief Tchatka.

Tchatka, who was both a chief and a medicine man, was born in the early 1770s. He was described by one observer as a "queer kind of grizzly bear fellow, very odd in his nature" and "the terror of neighboring tribes." He had unified several Assiniboin bands, and he claimed to be guided by *wak-kons*, or sacred spirits.

Because of their wide range of movement and nomadic ways, some bands of the Assiniboin tribe also traded at Fort Union.

Established in 1830, Fort Union was located at the mouth of the Yellowstone River—farther north into Indian country than Fort Clark and nearly eighteen hundred miles upriver of Saint Louis. Visitors arriving by boat or birchbark canoe would edge up against the riverbank, step over a muddy plank, and come face-to-face with the huge double doors of the fort.

A daunting structure, Fort Union was built to handle the heavy volume of goods from trade with tribes west of the fort. The fort was actually a compound protected by walls of cottonwood logs reaching twenty feet high, punctuated here and there by cannons loaded for action. Its large area held handsome living quarters, storage rooms, and a busy kitchen and dining room. The fort also housed a milk house and dairy and shops for coopers, tinsmiths, and gunsmiths. One of the shopkeepers, Charles Larpenteur, kept a daily journal of the comings and go-

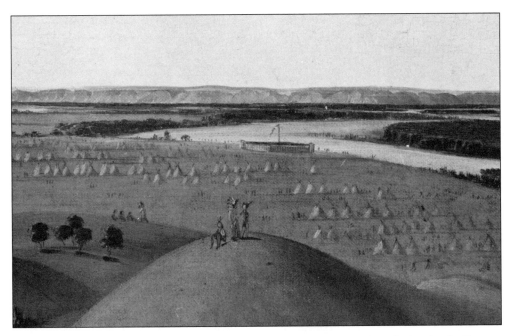

Fort Union, established in 1830, was an important center of trade for the Indian tribes that lived by the fort.

15

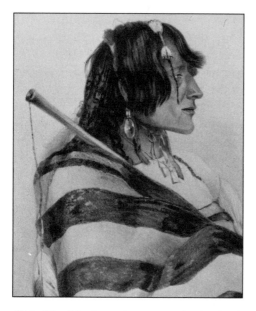

This Blackfoot warrior wears the typical garments of the Piegan group. The Blackfoot were experts on horseback.

ings at the fort. Larpenteur knew many of the Assiniboin as well as members of the newer trading partners, such as the Blackfoot.

The Blackfoot

Next to the Sioux Indians, who were also known as the Dakota or Lakota, the Blackfoot were the largest and most warlike tribe on the plains. They were also one of the Assiniboin's most dangerous enemies. The Blackfoot were masters of the horse, which they used for buffalo hunting and war. Legend says that their name refers to the blackening of the soles of their moccasins by the ashes of a prairie fire.

The Blackfoot were divided into three subgroups: the Blackfoot proper, the Bloods, and the Piegan. Their range extended from the plains of Montana to the Rocky Mountains, which they called "the backbone of the land."

The Blackfoot traded at Fort McKenzie, several days' journey up the river from Fort Union. Established in 1832, Fort McKenzie was located about six miles above the Marias River, a tributary of the Yellowstone River, which fed into the Missouri. The fort was led by Commander Alexander Culbertson, a burly man who was married to a Blackfoot squaw. By the mid-1830s, the banks of the river upon which Fort McKenzie sat usually held the tepees of many Blackfoot, Piegan, and Blood Indians who had interrupted warfare with other tribes— and among themselves—to trade.

In the 1830s, Ninoch-Kiaiu (Bear Chief) and Mehkshehme-Sukahs (Iron Shirt) were the great leaders of the Blackfoot. Bear Chief had a large, crooked nose and long hair that swept down over his face, and he wore a felt hat with a brass rim. As chief, he would organize trade with the American Fur Company's representatives at Fort McKenzie.

Horse Stealing and War

When not engaged in trade, Blackfoot warriors often stole horses from their neighbors, such as the Assiniboin. Horses were valuable possessions but hard to acquire. The Blackfoot warriors had to ride into the heart of the enemy camp to get the horses, which were always tethered and guarded. These attempts required both recklessness and athletic skill on the part of the young

Blackfoot men who regarded it as sport.

Horse stealing would often lead the Blackfoot into battle. First, a band of perhaps one hundred warriors would set out at night toward the enemy camp. After settling in at the edge of the camp, the surprise attack would be launched. The attackers favored hit-and-run tactics over hand-to-hand combat. Battles were fought on horseback, using short bows, hatchets, knives—and later rifles—as weapons. Ten or twenty from each side might die in a war, and each death was considered a tragedy by the surviving warriors.

The Blackfoot tribe would also wage war simply for sport. War was in one sense a pastime or game, and it could be called off if the fighting grew too fierce. The Blackfoot often had an understanding with their enemies that they would not inflict terrible harm. Prisoners were usually treated well. In victory, the Blackfoot would often adopt the Assiniboin warriors instead of torturing and killing them.

In battle, Blackfoot warriors acquired points for each act of bravery, which improved their reputation in the tribe. For some tribes, more points were gained by touch-

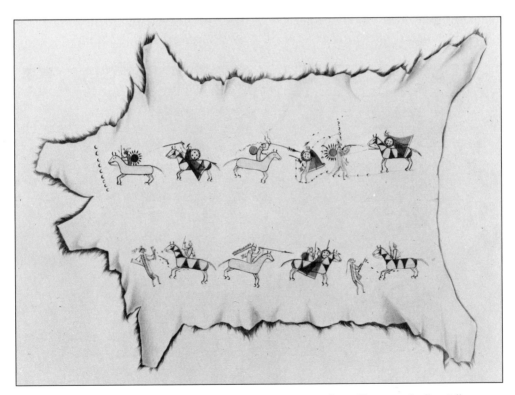

This buffalo robe depicts a battle between two warriors. To many Indian tribes, waging war served many purposes. The Blackfoot often waged war as a pastime or game.

ing a live enemy with a stick than by killing him.

But Indian battles could be horrible, too. James Beckwourth, a black frontiersman, witnessed one such battle where there was no mutual understanding between the tribes: "The clash of battle-axes, and the yells of the opposing combatants were truly appalling. . . . The blood [of the wounded] formed a pool which emitted a sickening smell as the warm vapor ascended to our nostrils. . . . Victims who were making away with their bowels ripped open were instantly felled with the battle-axe and stilled in death."

In their burial ceremonies, the Blackfoot placed the body on a scaffold constructed high in a tree and protected by thorns to discourage animals. After the body had deteriorated and the scaffold had fallen down, the bones of the deceased were buried in a special spot either on the prairie or along a riverbank. The skull of the deceased was buried with others in a separate, special burial area.

To Indians all over the country, the afterlife was a "happy hunting ground," open to all who died, even those who had not lived a virtuous life on earth. In the afterlife, one was reunited with friends and relatives. Some Indian tribes did not have a detailed system of belief about what the afterlife involved; they preferred to think about this world rather than the next.

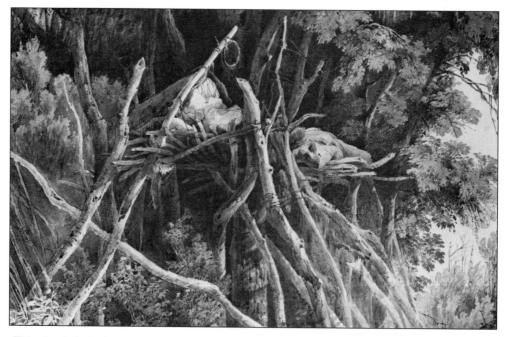

This Assiniboin burial scaffold is similar to the method used by other Plains Indians. After the scaffold and body decay and fall to the ground, the body is buried in a special burial ground.

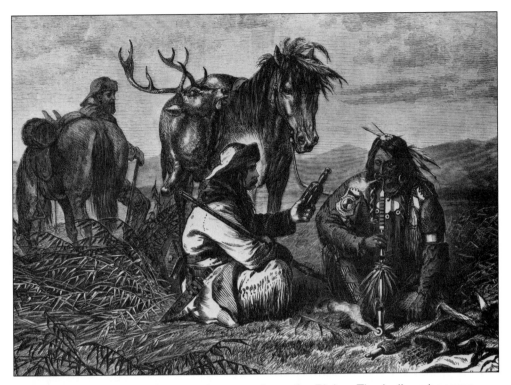

An Indian and a settler negotiate a trade on the Plains. The Indians became dependent on whites for certain goods, including knives, guns, ammunition, and alcohol.

In the world of the Plains Indians of the 1830s, the white settlers began to gain importance. The whites had given the Indians guns, cloth, utensils, and also alcohol, which was highly valued for its intoxicating effects. The Indians began to become dependent on the whites for these goods. Especially in times of drought or famine, the Indians anxiously awaited the arrival of the traders. Though they had prospered for generations before ever even seeing the white settlers, the Indians began to feel that these products they received through trade were necessary to their survival.

Through contact with white settlers and their goods, Indian culture changed. Alcohol was abused by many Indians and led some of them into alcoholism. Guns changed warfare for the Indians by making the fighting far more deadly. Whites also brought new contagious diseases to the Indians. The Indians were a remarkably healthy people and suffered from few natural diseases before contact with whites. Scurvy, tuberculosis, measles, cholera, typhoid—all were unknown before whites arrived. All of these diseases became feared killers among the tribes. The most feared, however, was smallpox.

1782 killed about 130,000 Indians. One out of every 4 members of virtually every tribe among the Plains Indians died. In the plague of 1801 and 1802, communities from the Plains states to Louisiana were ravaged and destroyed. In 1830, another plague struck, and the Mandan in particular suffered a devastating loss—about 1,500 members, or nearly half their tribe. The Assiniboin, Blackfoot, and other tribes of the upper Missouri River had all suffered over the years from smallpox, too.

Two

Smallpox and the Indians

Although smallpox was not a disease native to North America, the Indians had much experience with it. The Spaniards brought the disease to the Caribbean islands, Florida, and Mexico in the 1600s. Since that time, the disease periodically crept north and up the eastern coast, destroying Indian communities in its path.

Between 1616 and 1619, a great plague along the Massachusetts coast killed more than 90 percent of the Indian population in that area, including the Narragansett tribe. Only ten years later, smallpox in the Saint Lawrence region of eastern Canada killed tens of thousands of Iroquois. A century later, smallpox reduced the Cherokee population by half.

The great plague of 1781 and

Smallpox

Known to the world for centuries, smallpox has been one of humanity's greatest afflictions. Researcher Allan Chase claims, "All things being equal, in terms of the sheer numbers of people killed, blinded, crippled, pitted, and scarred by smallpox for at least two thousand years of oral and written history, this disease was most probably the worst pestilence ever to afflict humankind."

Like measles, smallpox is caused by an infectious virus. A virus is a tiny parasite that attacks and inhabits healthy cells without killing them. Then the virus forces these cells to produce more viruses. As these viruses multiply, they may eventually take over the whole body.

Smallpox is transmitted through physical contact. A person can get the disease by touching an infected blanket or by breathing the air near a victim. About half of all people who come in contact with the virus

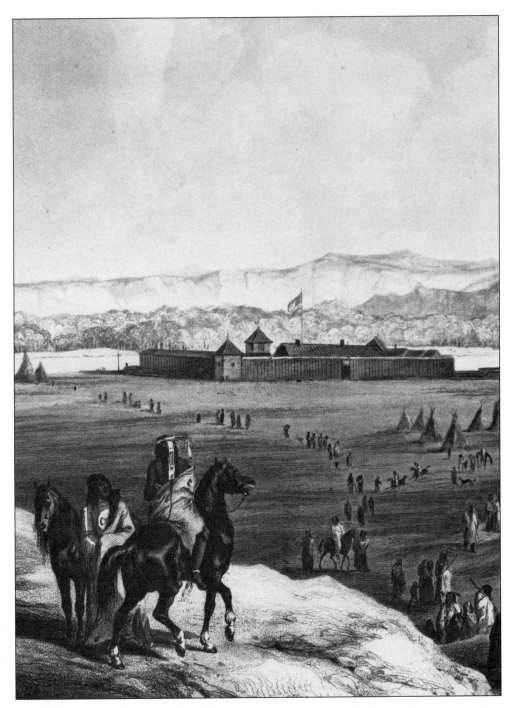

Indians approach Fort Union on the Missouri to trade crafts for metal goods and food. Many Indians were highly susceptible to smallpox and could catch it easily from infected whites—even from blankets or clothing.

THE DISCOVERY OF SMALLPOX VACCINE

In 1716, Lady Mary Wortley Montagu, the wife of the British ambassador to Turkey, observed inoculation procedures in Turkey. She watched as fifteen or twenty members of a community were inoculated and then confined to a small house for several weeks. The infections that developed were mild, and soon the inoculated members were allowed to return to their communities.

Lady Montagu convinced the royal family in Great Britain of the benefits of inoculation. The technique was first used on prisoners, then on members of the royal family. By the 1720s, inoculation was an accepted technique for some doctors in Britain. Twenty-five years later, the Smallpox and Inoculation Hospital was established in England, and the inoculation technique was further refined.

Though used throughout the eighteenth century, smallpox inoculation had its disadvantages. Those undergoing the procedure were very contagious and had to be quarantined to prevent others in the community from catching the virus. Also, patients almost always suffered from scarred skin, and sometimes the implanted virus was more dangerous in certain patients than anticipated. Many people died.

But inoculation was the only choice people had in the face of an epidemic. It saved many lives and in 1776 even helped win a battle. British soldiers, outnumbered three to one by the American colonial army in Quebec, Canada, were victorious over the smallpox-ravaged Americans. The British soldiers had undergone the inoculation technique and were immune from smallpox, but the American soldiers caught it and suffered. After the defeat at Quebec, Congress ordered inoculation for members of the military.

In 1796, an Englishman named Edward Jenner discovered the use of vaccination against smallpox. Jenner, a country doctor, observed that women

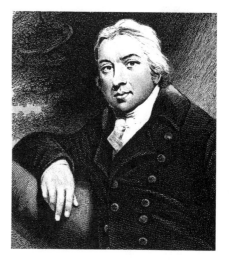

Edward Jenner discovered the smallpox vaccine in 1796.

who milked cows often caught cowpox, a mild virus related to smallpox that infected cows. The milkmaids seemed immune to the smallpox that routinely struck rural England. On May 14, 1796, Jenner took material from a cowpox sore on the hand of a milkmaid and transferred it to the arm of a healthy eight-year-old boy. The boy was mildly ill from the cowpox virus for about three days, and then his health returned. Jenner then tried to infect the boy with smallpox virus, but the virus did not harm him. The boy was immune to it.

After two years of successful experiments with other patients, Jenner announced his discovery of a way to make people immune from smallpox without first exposing them to the disease. In a text he published himself, titled *An Inquiry into the Causes and Effects of the Variolae Vaccinae*, Jenner coined the term *vaccination* and explained how it worked. Other doctors began to use Jenner's methods, and by 1801 more than 100,000 British citizens had been vaccinated.

become infected.

Once contracted, smallpox follows an established course. The patient becomes ill between seven and seventeen days after exposure to a person with the virus. First, there is fever, then an aching in the back. A rash then appears, which lasts about two days. Papules, or pimples, replace the rash. They are usually more numerous on the face, arms, and legs. At this stage, smallpox may be mistaken for chicken pox or measles. After four or five days, the papules become pustules, which are larger bumps containing pus. After a week, the pustules dry up and dark scabs form over them. At the end of two weeks, the scabs fall off, leaving pink spots on the skin. Until all the scabs fall off, the patient may still spread infection.

There are various forms of pox that are not smallpox but can affect humans. These other forms include chicken pox, monkey pox, buffalo pox, and cowpox. Like smallpox, they all produce pocks, or bumps, on the skin.

Four Smallpox Viruses

There are four viruses associated with smallpox. The first three are known as variola virus and include variola minor, variola intermedia (sometimes called the African strain), and the deadliest virus—variola major. Those infected with variola major suffer terribly. The infected skin, which smells horrible, looks like it has been burned or scalded, and the infected person feels like he or she is on fire. The disease kills by attacking the heart, liver, and lungs. Patients with this most severe form die when blood vessels burst as a result of the disease.

Vaccinia, the fourth virus, is less harmful than the others and is used in smallpox vaccines. In vaccination, a less fatal form of the virus is given to a patient by an injection. The similar virus can give the person a mild form of the disease. The person's immune system then creates antibodies to fight it off. Antibodies are substances produced by the body to kill bacteria, viruses, and other germs that cause disease. After destroying the virus, the antibodies remain permanently in the body and are capable of resisting any future attack by more deadly forms of the virus.

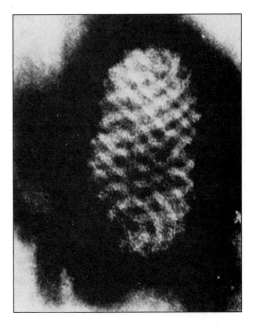

Smallpox is caused by a virus, a tiny parasite.

Before the invention of vaccines, the only way to become immune to smallpox was to survive an attack of it. Then the body possessed the proper antibodies to fight off a future attack. But those who lived through an attack of smallpox often suffered from scars and blindness. Many more did not survive at all. It is estimated that throughout history, one in four victims of smallpox has died. This number is even higher for the Indians.

Susceptibility

North American Indians were particularly susceptible to the smallpox virus. During the first half of the nineteenth century, whites offered many false reasons for why this was true. One observer decided that because Indian homes of buffalo hides were very exposed to the elements, Indians were too worn out from fighting the elements to be able to fight off disease. It was also suggested that the Indian diet, which was dominated by meat, somehow caused them to come down with smallpox more easily.

It is now known that, except for those tribal elders who had survived previous epidemics, most North American Indians had never been in contact with smallpox or any virus similar to it. Therefore, they had not developed the antibodies needed to fight off the smallpox virus.

This lack of exposure seems to explain why the Indians always caught the worst form of smallpox—variola major, or hemorrhagic smallpox. One writer, noting that the Indians often caught the most deadly strain, declared the disease to be "the natural curse of the red man."

Disease Spread Rapidly

Once the Indians contracted smallpox, the disease spread rapidly among them. The tribal villages

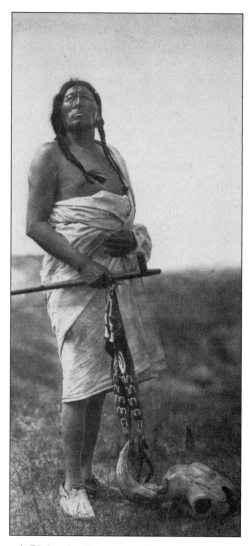

A Plains Indian poses for the camera. Whites had many opinions on why Indians contracted smallpox, most of them based on racism.

24

were often crowded, with tepees or lodges right up against one another and families living wall to wall. This closeness allowed the disease to travel easily. The disease also spread when some tribes tried to outrun it. Often, tribes without enemies on their borders would abandon their homes and usually spread the disease to their neighbors. Once infected, the Indians attempted to cure themselves by consulting the tribal medicine man, sometimes with disastrous results. Because the medicine men had very little knowledge of diseases, they often thought of cures that were worse than, or of methods that spread, rather than cured, the disease. In one technique, Indians tried to scare away the evil spirits they thought were causing the disease. A healthy Indian would stay with the infected person and act bravely. Instead of scaring away evil spirits, healthy members of the tribe would simply catch the disease.

Suspicions

Even though a smallpox vaccine did exist, the Indians were generally suspicious of the medicine, with good reason. Many knew that in some cases, smallpox had been purposely transmitted to them by white settlers to kill them off. Isaac McCoy confirmed in his 1836 *Annual of Indian Affairs* that settlers deliberately infected Indian tribes of the Southwest, including the Pawnee. Increase Mather, the colonial preacher and scholar who served as president of Harvard College, encouraged the spread of smallpox from settlers to

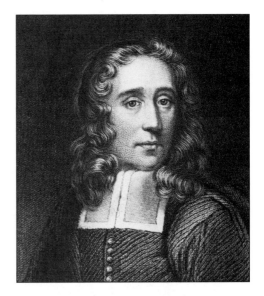

Some malicious settlers deliberately infected Indian tribes with the deadly smallpox. Increase Mather (above) was one colonist accused of doing so.

Indians through infected blankets. Mather did this in hopes that the Indians would die or move on, leaving the area open for American settlers. George Catlin summed up the feelings of the Indians about the vaccine: "They see white men urging the operation so earnestly they decide that it must be some new mode or trick of the pale face by which they hope to gain some new advantage over them."

The Indians were deathly afraid of any threats from the white settlers having to do with smallpox. James McDougal, a fur trader at Fort Astoria at the mouth of the Columbia River, knew this well. When the fort was threatened with attack after a dispute between traders and local Chinook Indians in 1811 and 1812, McDougal called a meeting with

INOCULATION AND VACCINATION

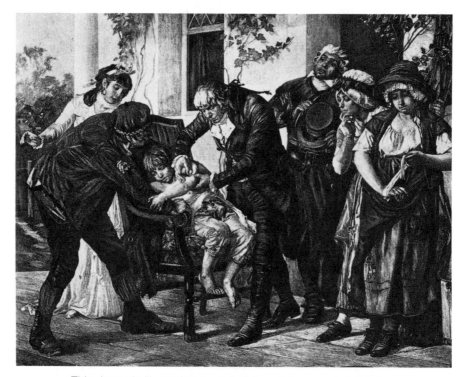

This dramatic illustration depicts Edward Jenner administering the first smallpox vaccination.

Inoculation is the deliberate infection of an individual with a mild strain of a disease to prevent a future, more deadly version of that same infection. Inoculation has been used throughout history to prevent smallpox. In ancient China, doctors blew dried and crushed smallpox scabs up the noses of patients to prevent the disease. This method worked in a good number of cases. In smallpox inoculation, the skin of a healthy patient is opened and bits of matter from smallpox scabs from a mild case of smallpox are inserted. This practice began in the Orient thousands of years ago and continued to be used until the end of the eighteenth century.

In this type of inoculation, the patient becomes mildly ill and is put under quarantine for two or three weeks as the body fights off the smallpox virus. The patient's body produces antibodies, which attack and destroy specific germs. The antibodies encircle the infected cells, making it difficult for the virus to spread, and soon the virus dies. After the viral attack, the antibodies stay in the body, ready to ward off any new attack.

Modern smallpox vaccination does not involve the smallpox virus at all. Instead, the cowpox virus is used, and it has almost no ill effects on humans. The healthy patient is injected with the cowpox virus, taken from the skin of an infected cow. After several days of fighting the virus, the body produces antibodies that are able to fight both cowpox and smallpox, which are very similar viruses. Vaccination replaced inoculation as a defense against smallpox.

Chinook leaders. At the meeting, he suddenly pulled a bottle from his bag and held it up high. "Listen: I am the smallpox chief. In this bottle I have it confined. All I have to do is to pull the cork, send it forth among you, and you are dead men," McDougal told them. This tactic deterred the Indians. They cancelled the planned attack on Fort Astoria.

In the early 1800s, the U.S. government did not consider vaccination programs for Indians a priority. After a terrible smallpox plague among the Southwestern tribes in 1815 and 1816, in which the Comanche alone lost four thousand people, local observer W.A. Trimble made earnest recommendations to Secretary of War John Calhoun that the Indians be immunized. These recommendations were ignored.

Some concerned settlers took vaccination into their own hands. After a severe plague in California in 1828, an adventurer named James Pattie claimed he personally vaccinated twenty-two thousand people, mostly California Indians who lived in Catholic missions. Though this figure is probably exaggerated, Pattie did perform vaccinations and protected many Indians from disease.

Congress Commits Funds

In 1832, Congress agreed to spend twelve thousand dollars to begin vaccinating the Indians. The money was to pay for physicians and the purchase of vaccines. Some success resulted. But for the most part, vaccination programs for Indians in

OPPOSITION

Edward Jenner's vaccination techniques would not be accepted by governments around the world for one hundred years. His discovery was ignored or suppressed for a variety of reasons. Leaders in France and Great Britain actually wanted the lower classes, who made up the labor force, to catch diseases so their populations did not increase. Political and business leaders thought that as long as workers' lives were disrupted by disease, suffering, and death, the workers would be too confused and hopeless to organize and rebel.

Policies against eradicating epidemics were also often supported by scholars. Soon after Jenner made his discovery, Thomas Malthus, a professor of political economy in England, wrote his famous *Essay on the Principle of Population*. In the essay, Malthus explained that an epidemic was a natural event that helped society get rid of its surplus poor, who "bred recklessly" and endangered an orderly society. Malthus further insisted that even if smallpox were eradicated, other diseases would appear to wipe out the poor. This was simply nature's way of reducing a population that has grown too large.

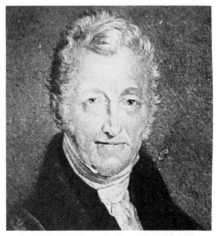

Thomas Malthus believed epidemics were a form of population control.

the first part of the nineteenth century either failed or were never started.

One reason for this failure was the unavailability of the vaccine. Difficult to find in the cities, the vaccine was nearly impossible to find at the forts and on the frontier. There were not many doctors or scientists who believed in the vaccine and knew whom to get it from or how to manufacture it. Many doctors had experience with bad or weak vaccine that was ineffective. This led them to doubt the entire idea of vaccination. If brought upriver during an epidemic, the precious medicine would go first to any white settlers who wanted it—and most of them did.

Useless Vaccine

Due to contamination or improper methods of preservation, many samples of vaccine that did arrive safely at the forts were useless anyway. Sometimes, vaccine would arrive infected with bacteria, which was passed on to patients. Terrible illness and death could result. Doctors did not discover proper preservation and refrigeration techniques until the twentieth century.

Even when the vaccine arrived on the frontier in good condition, there were not enough physicians to administer it. The federal government had a hard time finding doctors willing to leave the comfort and safety of the cities and small towns for the unknown of the wilderness. As a result, most vaccinations performed on Indians were performed

by anyone who knew how to hold a syringe. Severe infections often resulted from improper injections. One settler described these efforts: "It has been practiced only during the last few years by amateurs for up to the present date there is no physician in the whole territory."

The lack of communication between cities and the frontier also prevented vaccine from reaching Indians or settlers. No white settlements existed in the vast wilderness except for the trading posts dotting the banks of the larger rivers. A letter pleading for vaccine would take at least four months to get from Fort

THE TARBOROUGH AFFAIR

The Tarborough Affair probably kept a national vaccine program from taking hold in the United States in the first half of the nineteenth century. In 1813, Congress established a national vaccine agency with Dr. James Smith as its director. Smith had been directing the nation's first vaccine institute in Baltimore since 1802. Through the new agency, Smith hoped to make vaccination more appealing and more accessible to Americans.

On November 1, 1821, Smith made a tragic mistake. He mailed smallpox scabs, which contained deadly smallpox virus, instead of cowpox vaccine to a vaccinator in Tarborough, North Carolina. Two months later came the terrible news—Smith's "vaccine" had, in fact, caused smallpox in Tarborough, and several people had died. Though Smith claimed innocence, a whole nation panicked. People were more scared of vaccination than the disease itself. The Tarborough Affair resulted in the repeal of Smith's National Vaccine Agency, which closed one year after the affair.

Clark to Saint Louis. In four months, whole tribes might be dead.

In the first half of the nineteenth century, white indifference toward Indians was another problem that prevented the establishment of vaccination programs. The highest priority of the settlers was to establish settlements in the hostile wilderness—not to save lives of the hostile Indians. The federal government was of no help. Federal funds were spent on building forts for settlements, not providing vaccine for those who made settlement difficult.

Trading Continues

Despite suspicion and conflict between whites and Indians, trade between them thrived in the early 1830s, especially on the upper Missouri River. At the beginning of the decade, a contract was signed between the Assiniboin, Blackfoot, and the American Fur Company, binding them in trade. At that time, the Mandan and American Fur were already partners and were benefiting from trade.

A Difficult Winter

But in June 1837, the Mandan were in bad shape. It had been a difficult winter. Their crop yield had been poor. Much of the Mandan tribe was malnourished, and many had already died of starvation. Mato-toh-pah's braves had not gathered many furs because of recent wars with the Sioux. That year, the buffalo herds were far away on the plains, and the Mandan, who were limited in their hunting range by the Sioux, were forced to fight. The hungry Mandan warriors spent the days searching for buffalo and any other food they could find as they awaited the summer arrival of the American Fur Company's steamship.

Three

The Destroying Angel

In June 1937, the American Fur Company's steamboat, called the *St. Peter*, was forging up the Missouri River on its yearly trip from Saint Louis. The river was so low that the boat had difficulty getting through. Sixty miles south of Fort Clark, while at a trading post called the Blacksnake Hills, a crew member became ill with smallpox. First came fever, then pustules. American Fur officials knew what a devastating effect the disease could have on the Indians they would contact. Still, they did not put the man ashore to prevent contaminating the Indians upriver. Continuing its journey, the *St. Peter* did meet up with members of the Sioux tribe, and boatmen warned them of the disease on board. Though sorry to lose the opportunity to trade, the Sioux wisely returned to the prairie.

It is hard to imagine that the traders of the American Fur Company did not take precautions to keep smallpox away from the Indians. Smallpox could have brought an end to the lucrative trade with the Indians. But the company did not want to lose any sailors during the busy trading season. Within days, a few others became ill, and the disease was diagnosed as smallpox. But the *St. Peter* continued on toward Fort Clark and the Mandan villages.

On June 19, the *St. Peter* arrived at Fort Clark. Trading began immediately after the Mandan returned from their buffalo hunt. For two full days, Indians and whites mixed freely, trading pelts, tobacco, and copper utensils. When business was through, the *St. Peter* continued up the river. No one among the Mandan suspected that the steamship had brought the deadly smallpox virus with it.

Source of Infection Unknown

Exactly how the Mandan became infected with smallpox is unknown. According to legend, one of the Mandan chiefs stole a blanket from the *St. Peter*. F. A. Chardon, in charge at the fort, observed what happened. Chardon realized that this particular blanket had been used by an ill ship hand and was probably infected. Chardon and the ship's captain tried to convince the Indian chief to return the blanket at once. The chief would be pardoned for his crime, and the trappers would even

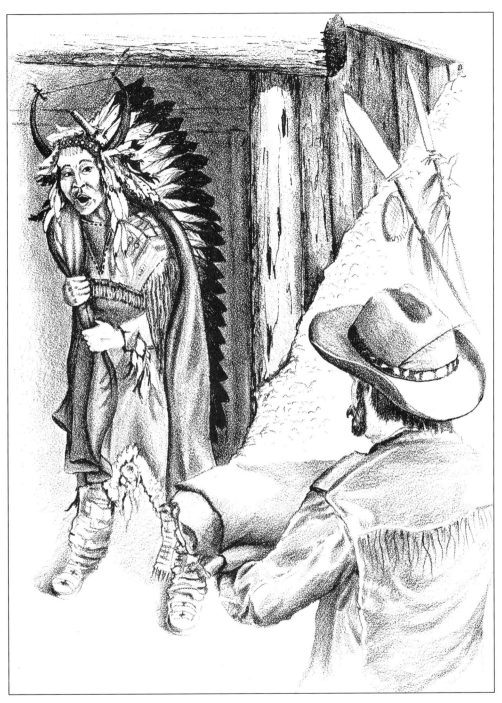

F.A. Chardon tries to convince a Mandan chief to relinquish a blanket infected with the deadly smallpox. According to legend, the stolen blanket caused the terrible epidemic among the Mandan.

give him other blankets in return for the infected one. But the chief refused, and the stolen blanket remained with the Mandan.

On Friday, July 14, about three weeks after the *St. Peter* had departed, the first death among the Mandan occurred at Fort Clark. "A young Mandan died today of the smallpox," reported Commander Chardon. "Several others have caught it." Over the weekend, several more cases were reported.

Soon, the suffering was widespread. The smallpox virus worked its way through the tribe quickly and effectively. A horrified Chardon reported that "the patient, when first seized, complains of dreadful pains in the head and back, and in a few hours he is dead: the body immediately turns black, and swells to thrice its natural size."

Within days, Chief Ma-to-toh-pah also caught the pox. The great Mandan leader had always insisted that his tribe benefited from contact with the settlers. Now, though, Ma-to-toh-pah was convinced he had been wrong. In what was probably his last speech to his tribespeople, Ma-to-toh-pah expressed his anger at the white settlers: "I have never called a white man a dog, but today I do pronounce them to be a set of black-hearted dogs, they have deceived me, them that I always considered as brothers, has turned out to be my worst enemies. . . . I do not fear death, my friends. You know it, but

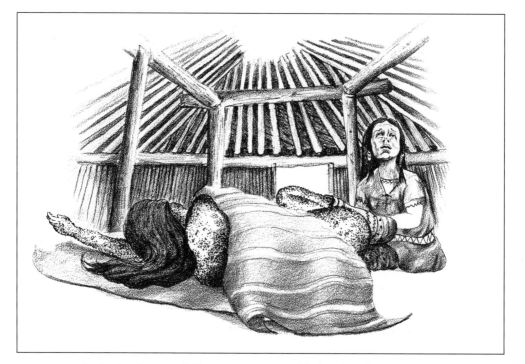

An Indian keeps vigil over a woman with the deadly smallpox.

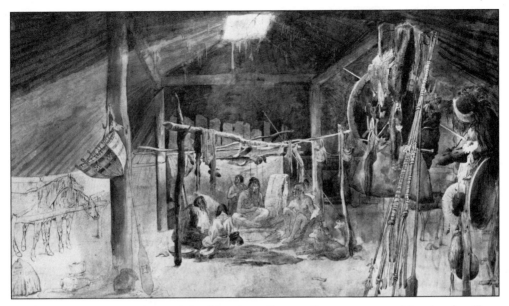

Smallpox quickly devastated the Mandan villages. Because many Mandan families lived closely together in earth lodges, the disease spread quickly.

to die with my face rotten, that even the wolves will shrink with horror at seeing me, and say to themselves, that is the Four Bears, the Friend of the Whites."

The day after Ma-to-toh-pah's speech, Chardon reported that "the smallpox is killing them up at the village, four died today." The Mandan, he said, "are getting worse. . . . Where the disease will stop, I know not."

The next few weeks saw no end to the tragedy. Chardon wrote, "A Mandan and his wife killed themselves yesterday, to not outlive their relations that are dead." The following day, he recorded this horrible event: "The wife of a young Mandan that caught the disease was suffering from the pain, her husband looked at her, and held down his head. He jumped up, and said to his wife,

When you were young, you were handsome, you are now ugly and going to leave me, but no, I will go with you. He took up his gun and shot her dead, and with his knife ripped open his own belly."

Death swarmed over the Mandan villages. One brave cut his own throat. Another suffering brave forced an arrow down his throat and into his lungs. A squaw who had watched her husband suffer and die hanged her children and shot herself. A son asked his mother to help him dig a grave, and then the boy, with his father's help, lay down and died in it.

These and other grief-struck Indians took their own lives because they could not bear to wait for death to take them as it had taken their family and friends. One observer recalled, "When they saw all their rela-

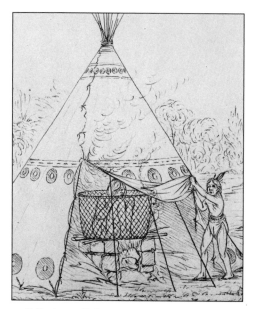

Tribal medicine men recommended alternating sweat baths and ice baths to cure the pox. Unfortunately, this procedure often resulted in hastening a victim's death.

rocks to produce a great amount of steam. After exposure to the steam, the patient hurried to the nearby river and plunged in. An untold number of infected Indians died this way when their systems were unable to withstand the shock.

Dreams Against the Virus

When the ice baths failed, the medicine men tried to help by interpreting the dreams of the victims. In dreams, an Indian could find warnings, prophecies, and revelations. Surely, if there were a way to fight off the invisible killer, it would be revealed in a dream. Medicine men tried to stimulate dreams among ill members of the tribe through fasting, dancing, and torture. Chardon reported, "Some of them have made dreams that they talked to the sun, others to the moon, several articles have been sacrificed to them both." Despite the revelations offered, though, dreams were no match for the deadly virus.

Desperate to save their loved ones from infection, Indians also tried to vaccinate themselves by applying smallpox scabs to the flesh of the healthy. In most cases, this method proved ineffective, though sometimes there was success. Chardon reported that an Indian vaccinated his own child "by cutting two small pieces of flesh out of his arms, and two on the belly, and then taking a scab from one . . . and rubbing it on the wounded part . . . three days later the child is well."

Some Indians were just lucky. Chardon created a cure for one In-

tions buried, and the pestilence still raging with unabated fury about the remainder of their countrymen, life became a burden to them, and they put an end to their wretched existence, either with their knives and muskets, or by precipitating themselves from the summit of the rock near their settlement." Catlin, who was a friend to the Mandan, in anguish summarized the disaster at the villages: "They destroyed themselves."

The Medicine Men

The medicine men, or healers, did their best to help. First, they tried using alternating sweat baths and ice baths. Those with the pox were put inside a special tepee, where water was poured over heated dian, supplying him with a mixture of magnesia, peppermint, and sugar—"all mixed together . . . with Indian grog"—and claimed that the concoction worked, adding that he believed positive thinking had a lot to do with the cure. He also gave six pounds of Epsom salts in doses to the victims' families but did not report on the effects.

Cured Themselves

In a few instances, Indians desperate for an end to their suffering cured themselves. Chardon reported that a young brave alone in his lodge was in so much pain that he wanted to die, so he began "to rub the scabs until blood was running all over his body." Then he rolled in the ashes of his fire, burning himself terribly, and two days later he was "perfectly well." Chardon also noted that few Indians desired to try this method.

The Death of Ma-to-toh-pah

Chief Ma-to-toh-pah, ill, watched from his lodge as everyone in his family died from the pox. What could the great man do now, facing such horror? With his wives and children all dead, Ma-to-toh-pah gathered up enough strength to walk through the village and weep at the destruction. Unclothed corpses

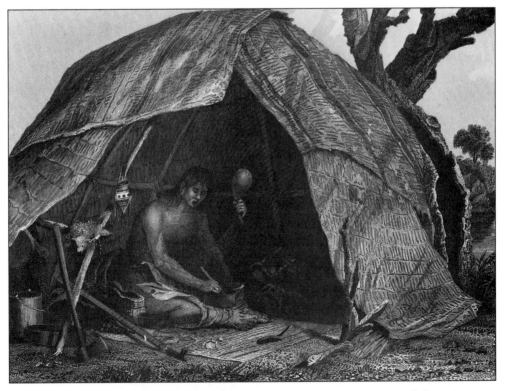

Medicine men tried other methods to cure smallpox. Here, a medicine man prepares a cure.

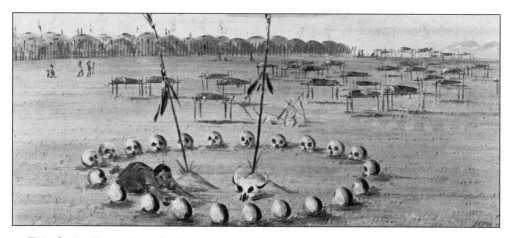

This Catlin illustration of a Mandan burial ground depicts a form of Indian burial. Note the corpses placed on scaffolds in the background. After the plague worsened, the Mandans could no longer maintain their traditional methods of burial.

lay swarming with flies in the doorways of the earth lodges, in the alleys between the buildings, and all around the stilled village.

Returning to his lodge, Ma-to-toh-pah gathered his family in a pile and covered them with buffalo robes. Then, determined to end his own suffering, he decided to starve himself to death. He left for a nearby hilltop and stayed there for six days without food or water, then crawled back to his lodge. He died on July 30, the ninth day of his starvation. His corpse lay in his lodge, along with the members of his family, all awaiting burial.

In previous plague years, burial had been performed according to the traditional manner. Now, there was no one to bury the dead. Corpses lay inside tepees or out in the village, along the paths that led to cornfields. Some corpses had a blanket thrown over them, but many were half-dressed or naked.

Wolves, dogs, and rats fed on the rotting flesh.

The white traders at Fort Clark had suffered, too, but the number of white victims was much lower. Many had accepted vaccination prior to their arrival at the fort, and those who had not been vaccinated proved to be fairly resistant to the disease. There were, in fact, no deaths recorded among the adults at Fort Clark, though the children were not as fortunate. "My youngest son died today," the weary Chardon reported on September 22.

By the end of September, the plague at Fort Clark had run its course. In the following year, a visitor to Mandan country reported: "The destroying angel has visited the unfortunate sons of the wilderness with terrors never before known, and has converted the extensive hunting grounds as well as the peaceful settlements of those tribes into desolate and boundless

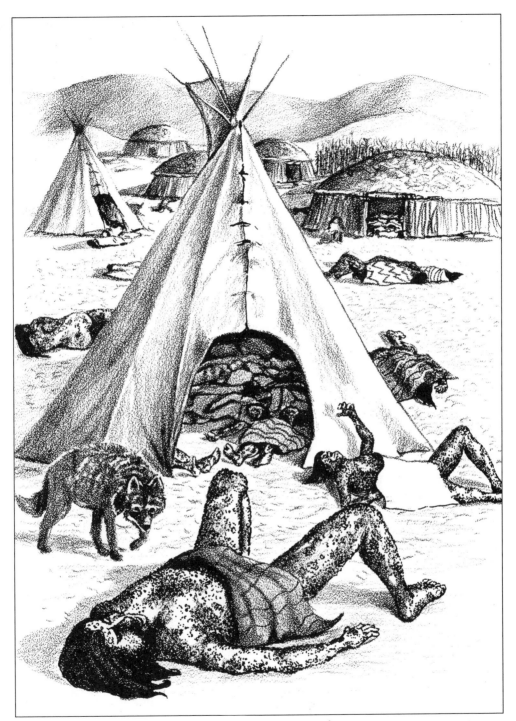

So many Mandan died from the smallpox that there was no one left to bury the dead. Corpses lay inside tepees or out in the village.

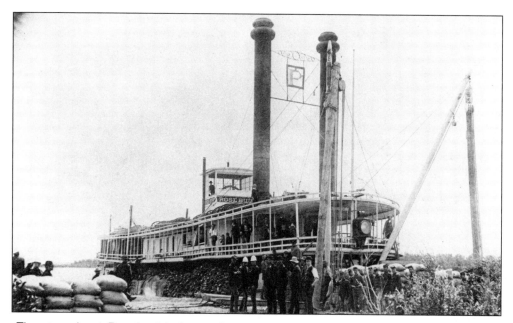

The steamboat *Rosebud* during a trip up the Missouri River. Crew members aboard a similar steamship, the *St. Peter*, passed the deadly smallpox virus to the Assiniboin tribe at Fort Union.

cemeteries." There had been about sixteen hundred members of the Mandan tribe before the plague struck in June 1837. Only thirty-one Mandan survived.

The Assiniboin at Fort Union

The smallpox plague, however, had only just begun with the Mandan. The *St. Peter* had continued on its fateful journey up the Missouri River, taking the awful smallpox virus with it.

The ship arrived at Fort Union in July. The white traders discovered that the Assiniboin tribe had camped out on the banks beside the fort. However, the Assiniboin men were out on a hunting trip. The crew of the steamship decided to wait a few days for the warriors to return. A trader aboard the *St. Peter*

named Jacob Halsey was now the carrier of the pox. He caught the virus from the ship hand who had infected the Mandan and then recovered. Halsey was quickly confined to the fort. Even so, a few whites and about thirty Assiniboin squaws who lived in the fort as wives of the resident Indian traders strayed close enough to Halsey to catch the disease.

Inoculation

With no vaccine available, the fort officials decided to try inoculation, or the injection of a small amount of virus into a healthy person in order to stimulate the immune system. Then, if the person later catches the disease, the body will have a good supply of antibodies able to fight it off. They used their medical reference book and called for Halsey. He had a mild case and allowed his skin to be used as inoculation material for the thirty squaws and a few white traders.

The results were disastrous. Instead of preventing smallpox, the inoculation procedure transmitted it. Some of those undergoing the procedure grew violently ill with what was certainly hemorrhagic smallpox and died within days, while the rest were confined to a room in the fort. The shopkeeper Charles Larpenteur described the inoculation survivors: "Some were half eaten by maggots, and some, in their delirium, were so crazed that they had to be locked in." Larpenteur also described the condition of the sick and dying: "There was such a stench in the fort that it could be smelt at the distance of 300 yards." It is believed that most of these initial victims of the virus at Fort Union died.

Suspicions Mounted

Meanwhile, the Assiniboin warriors returned from their hunting trip. Officials warned the men to stay away from the fort and its infected residents. The Assiniboin, though, were sure that the traders were just trying to manipulate them by postponing trading. Suspicions mounted because the Assiniboin were not allowed to see their thirty squaws. The Assiniboin chief, Tchatka, and his tribe remained in their camp just down the riverbank from the fort's entrance.

Days passed, and no entry was granted. The Indians were impa-

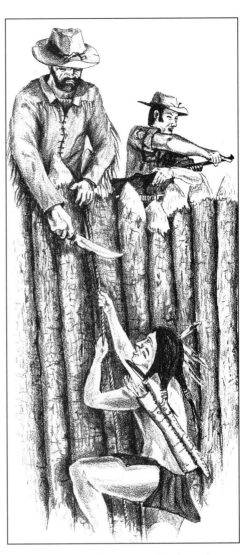

When denied entry to the fort, the Assiniboin became impatient. Some braves climbed the fort's walls in an attempt to steal horses.

tient with the excuses of the fort officials. Four or five braves climbed the fort's walls and tried to run a herd of horses out. Soldiers chased the braves and recaptured the horses, and in the close contact the virus was passed to the Indians.

39

A few days later, before the Assiniboin realized a few of their members had been infected, the smallpox virus was transmitted once again. Led by Tchatka, the warriors demanded entry to the fort. This time, they sought neither trade nor revenge; food supplies were low, and they were hungry. The epidemic inside was at its height. Even when warned of the dangers within, Tchatka would not back away from the huge double doors.

A Serious Situation

Desperate to convince the Assiniboin that the situation was serious, several officers went to the room where the sick were confined and brought out an infected boy. They walked him to the fort's entrance. They called for a group of warriors to approach and see for themselves the horror that lay inside the fort. The doors were swung wide open, and the Indians got a horrifying look at the boy's bloated, scab-ridden face. The doors were immediately swung shut again.

The Assiniboin warriors had been exposed to the infected boy for only a moment—but in that moment the smallpox was transmitted. Totally unaware that they were now infected, too, the Assiniboin warriors returned to their people, who were as yet untouched by the virus. The disease, however, quickly began to appear among them, and some bands tried to escape infection. Unlike the Mandan, many Assiniboin rode off, far away, and did avoid the plague. But the majority of Assiniboin caught the disease.

Death seemed to lie in wait for every Indian. One witness recalled that the Indians "died under corners of fences, in little groups, to which kindred ties held them in ghastly death, with their bodies swollen, and covered with pustules, their eyes blinded, hideously howling their death song in utter despair."

The Assiniboin believed that these deaths were purposely caused by whites. Tchatka and his warriors initially decided to avenge themselves, but soon their anger was overcome by hopelessness. Larpenteur observed, "The warlike spirit which . . . gave reason to apprehend the breaking out of a sanguinary war, is broken."

Most Assiniboin Succumb

The mortality rate among the Assiniboin was nearly 90 percent. It was reported that fifty to one hundred Assiniboin died every day. An anonymous letter writer reported: "I do not know how many Assiniboin have already died, as they have long since given up counting, but I presume at least 800." At least ten out of every twelve Assiniboin died, and the pestilence was still spreading.

The dead bodies of the Assiniboin remained unburied. Whole families lay in piles inside their homes, left to decay "and be devoured by their own dogs." A witness to the scene reported, "The mighty warriors are now the prey of the greedy wolves of the prairie, and the few survivors, in mute despair, throw themselves on the pity of the Whites, who, however, can do but little to help them."

The Blackfoot at Fort McKenzie

In mid-July, as the plague swept through the Assiniboin tribe, a small keelboat stocked with goods left Fort Union on its yearly trip west to Fort McKenzie. There, the whites would conduct their trade with the local Blackfoot Indians. The men who made the journey to Fort McKenzie were free of smallpox—or so they thought. In a matter of days, however, one crew member was diagnosed as having the disease.

The captain of the boat, Alexander Harvey, wanted to take every precaution to make sure that the disease would not spread to the Blackfoot waiting at Fort McKenzie. He stopped the boat downstream of the fort and sent word of the danger to his commander, Alexander Culbertson. Culbertson sent a message back to "stay with the cargo at the mouth of the Judith River until the disease passes."

Indians Insisted

Outside Fort McKenzie, a large number of Blood and Piegan Blackfoot awaited the boat's arrival. After a few days, they grew impatient and asked Culbertson what had happened. Culbertson explained that the boat was carrying disease. In-

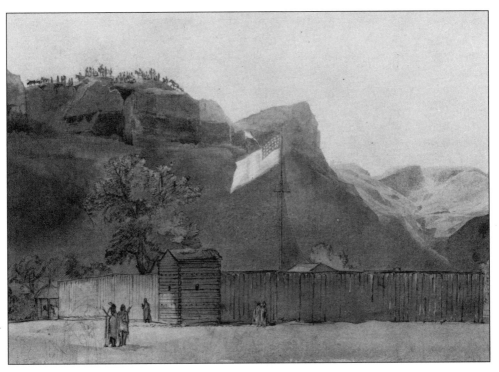

In mid-July, a small keelboat made its way to Fort McKenzie to trade with the Blackfoot tribe. The whites on the boat would carry the smallpox virus with them.

stead of resigning themselves to wait, the Blackfoot leaders demanded the boat be brought upstream. Culbertson protested, but the Indians insisted. If the order were not given, then they would go downstream to the boat, attack the crew, and seize the cargo.

Culbertson took the Blackfoot threats seriously. He sent word to Harvey to proceed with the journey. Soon, the boat arrived at Fort McKenzie, where trade was conducted as usual. After a few days, the Blackfoot left with their goods. There had been no sign of illness among them. Culbertson and his men were relieved.

The white soldiers became suspicious, however, when two months passed and no members of the Blackfoot tribe had been seen near the fort. It was the end of autumn now, and the Blackfoot should have already returned to trade for winter supplies. Culbertson set out one cold day with one of his men into the forest to look for the Indians.

The men arrived at Three Forks, where the Missouri River is formed from three other rivers and where the Blackfoot usually hunted beaver in the fall. But there was no sign of activity. They continued on through the frozen country to the Piegan village. There, they came upon a horrible sight. The sixty lodges in the village were deserted, and there were bodies everywhere. Trails of them led into the mountains. Birds

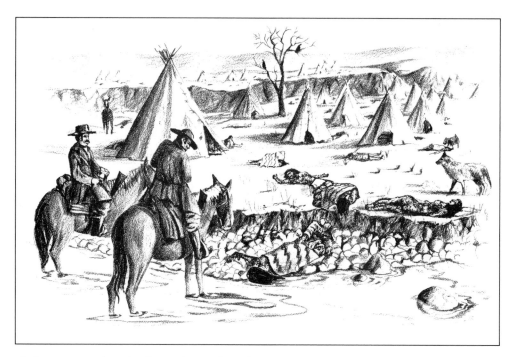

At least seven hundred members of the Blackfoot tribe died of smallpox. There were so many bodies that it was impossible to bury them all.

feasted on the corpses. The only survivors were two old women, murmuring death chants among the still bodies.

Burial was impossible because of the huge number of corpses and the bad weather. The soldiers thought it best to "collect the dead bodies and bury them in large pits; but since the ground is frozen we are obliged to throw them into the river."

One observer reported that at least seven hundred Blackfoot died near Fort McKenzie. In surrounding areas, as the disease wound its deadly trail, a total of six thousand—or two-thirds of the entire population of the Blackfoot, Piegan, and Bloods—perished.

Winter brought frost to the trees on the banks of the upper Missouri River. The hunting grounds of the Blackfoot, Mandan, and Assiniboin were quiet. Once alive with the activity of braves and squaws and children, the land was now a "vast field of death, covered with unburied corpses and spreading for miles, pestilence and infection," according to one observer.

Four

The Devastation Continues

From the tribes of the upper Missouri River, the plague traveled west, where almost no tribe escaped unscathed.

By October 1837, the Sioux were infected with smallpox, and in December, the Gros Ventres of Montana lost many members of their tribe. Next, the Crows caught it. In this year, the Indian tribes of New Mexico were also struck by smallpox.

The smallpox virus then spread south to California in late 1837, where it devastated various Indian tribes until 1839. In north-central California, it is estimated that smallpox killed three-fifths of the entire Indian population. A horrified witness described the scene: "No language can picture the scene of desolation which the country presents. In whatever direction we go, we see nothing but melancholy wrecks of human life. The tents are still standing on every hill, but no rising smoke announces the presence of human beings and no sounds but the croaking of the raven and the howling of the wolf interrupt the fearful silence."

The Indians of the Northwest coast saw the arrival of the plague in 1838, as did the Pawnee to the east. About two thousand of the ten thousand Pawnee perished. From the Pawnee, the disease traveled southwest to the Osage and the Kiowa. The Kiowan calendar calls the winter of 1839 and 1840 *Ta dalkop Sai*, (the smallpox winter).

The Chickasaw were the next victims, followed by the Choctaw and the Indian nations of the Arkansas River. In the spring of 1840, the plague struck the tribes of Texas and New Mexico, including the Comanche and Apache, before finally ending its course of death.

A whole continent of Indians had suffered terrible losses. George Catlin wrote in the aftermath of this devastation "of the numerous tribes which have already disappeared and of those that have been traded with up to the Rocky Mountains, each one had had this exotic disease in their turn, and in a few months have lost one-half or more of their numbers." It is estimated that 100,000 to 300,000 Indians died in the plague.

After the Plague

After the virus had destroyed their tribe, the remaining Blackfoot did not blame the whites for bring-

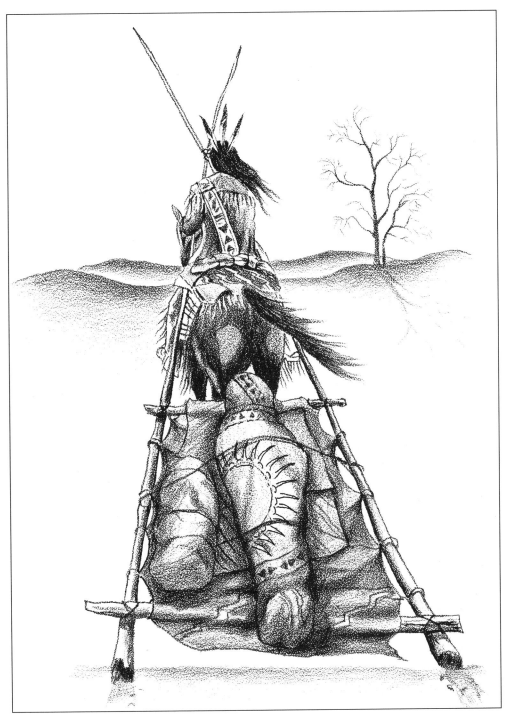

By 1840, a whole continent of Indians had suffered terrible losses from smallpox. It is estimated that 100,000 to 300,000 Indians died in the plague.

THE CALIFORNIA PLAGUE

In late 1837, at cavalry headquarters in Sonoma, California, Gen. Mariano Vallejo sent his corporal of cavalry, Ignacio Miramontes, west to Fort Ross on the coast for a cargo of cloth and leather goods. Returning to Sonoma with the goods, Miramontes unwittingly brought smallpox with him.

A large number of Indians at the Sonoma Mission, as well as many white men working as laborers at Vallejo's ranch, caught the disease. Vallejo tried to contain the disease—he even moved his entire ranch nearly two miles away—but his attempts were fruitless. The Indians "died daily like bugs."

The disease spread rapidly, killing off Indian populations "in the valleys of Sonoma, Petaluma, Santa Rosa, Russian River, Clear Lake, the Tulares [Sacramento] and extended to the slopes of Mount Shasta." The losses were catastrophic. In 1838, the peak year of this California plague, 200 whites, 3,000 mestizos (people of mixed European and Indian heritage), and 100,000 Indians were reported dead.

Though suffering severe losses, the Blackfoot population did survive and grow after the disaster. Within about seventeen years, it had regained all but one-third of its pre-plague population.

The Blackfoot tribe did not completely recover, however. Kinship ties had been destroyed. So many people had died that the survivors did not know whom children belonged to. Family relationships became confused. Cousins married cousins—and there were even innocent marriages between brother and sister. In 1870 and in the early 1880s, the Blackfoot again died in great numbers from smallpox plagues. Weakened by disease and helpless in the face of the disappearance of the buffalo on the prairies, the Blackfoot were no longer a mighty force on the northern plains. Under the strains of reservation life, their numbers decreased steadily until about 1900.

Of all the tribes affected, the Mandan probably suffered the most. Only thirty or forty people of the Mandan tribe survived the plague. Their neighbors the Arikara fared better, and after the plague fully subsided, the Arikara moved into the nearly deserted Mandan villages, which were built better than their own. Taking advantage of their new dominance, the Arikara took the surviving Mandan as slaves.

Cut to Pieces and Destroyed

The Arikara and their Mandan slaves lived for several relatively peaceful years, but peace was not to

ing the disease to them. Relations remained friendly between Culbertson's men and the Blackfoot for many years, though trading decreased as whites continued to encroach upon Blackfoot territory.

As the years passed, the Blackfoot tribes weakened. For the Blackfoot and most other tribes, the epidemic not only reduced their numbers, but seemed to kill those individuals who were most productive—adult men and women—while the very old and the very young were often the ones able to recuperate. It took years for the tribes to recover and for young members to grow into leaders.

last. The Arikara were finally attacked by the Sioux—the old enemy of the Mandan—and were badly outnumbered. The Sioux were bent on destroying the Arikara and the few Mandan that remained. Some Mandan saw the situation was hopeless and wanted to die. They ran into the prairie, yelling that they themselves were Arikara and that they wanted the Sioux to kill them because they had no family or friends left. As the Sioux approached, the Mandan fought furiously, and "they were thus cut to pieces and destroyed," said George Catlin.

By 1862, the many villages of the Mandan, Arikara, and the small Hidatsa tribe were combined into one village adjacent to the nearby and newly established Fort Berthold. Today, the descendants of the Mandan still live with their neighbors. There are no full-blooded Mandan left.

Only Eighty Escaped

The Assiniboin fared a little better than their neighbors, the Mandan. Many Assiniboin had fled during the epidemic. Chief Tchatka himself had been immunized by an earlier plague and did not die from the smallpox, but he now saw the end of his reign. Only eighty members of his band escaped with their lives. Tchatka died several years later in obscurity. At the end of the century, the remaining members of the once-powerful Assiniboin Indians were settled on reservations in Montana and Alberta, Canada.

The smallpox plague had caused many Indians to lose faith in their traditional way of life. Their medicine men had been completely ineffective against the invisible killer. The helplessness of their healers made the Indians bitter and skeptical. If they could not depend on their tribal wisdom and traditions to save them, what could they believe in? Their sense of control over their destiny had been shattered.

Little Outside Help

During the plague that lasted from 1837 to 1840, few outside efforts were made to vaccinate the Plains Indians. The commissioner of Indian Affairs, reporting from Wash-

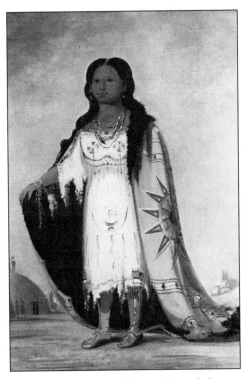

A young Arikara girl in traditional dress. The Arikara tribe was almost completely wiped out by smallpox.

ington at the time, claimed that "every exertion was made to confine the diseased, and much was done . . . to arrest the ravages by use of vaccination." Specifically, the commissioner claimed that a physician was sent with vaccine to the Columbia River area in the Northwest. But this token effort was made during the final period of the epidemic, after so many lives had already been lost.

Hoping They Would Disappear

After the plague, Plains Indians continued to receive little meaningful assistance from the federal government. The government was preoccupied with other problems, including trying to remove the Indi-

ans east of the Mississippi River to make room for white settlers. The Indians of the Plains were ignored. As the years passed, various local government positions were not filled. Little contact, good or bad, was initiated by the Bureau of Indian Affairs, which was supposed to be involved in tribal affairs throughout the nation. It seemed as if the federal government was hoping the Plains Indians would disappear so that their lands could be claimed.

Business Continued to Boom

Nor did the American Fur Company come to the aid of the Mandan, Assiniboin, and Blackfoot. At the time of the plague, officials of the American Fur Company had expected a great decline in profits. But this was not to be the case. Even though "our most profitable Indians have died," as one official put it, business continued to boom because the company was able to find other trading partners. Farther north, the Algonquin Cree, who had been naturally immunized against this plague by previous plagues, stepped into the range abandoned by the Assiniboin. The Cree became the dominant tribe in that northern region and the new partners of the American Fur Company. Because trade did not suffer, the company had no need to save its previous partners.

Smallpox continued to plague the Indians of North America until mid-century. The disease periodically reemerged with deadly force. The Indians of the Columbia River in

Washington and Oregon were struck by it in 1846. In 1848, the Iowa Indians, a Siouan-speaking tribe living in what is now Iowa, lost one hundred warriors and an uncounted number of women and children to smallpox. In 1850, the plague wiped out entire camps of the Cour d'Allene, as well as the Dakota. At this time, too, the Indians of the Aleutian Islands were struck by the disease.

The Homestead Act

Despite the ravages of smallpox, the Plains Indians dominated their range until mid-century. Until that time, white settlers were not very interested in living in the unfriendly wilderness. But along with the establishment of the Oregon Trail in the 1840s came forts along the trail to protect travelers. In 1865, as the Civil War ended, dispatched soldiers and new immigrants from Europe rushed out to the frontier to take advantage of the Homestead Act of 1862, which allowed a settler to claim a parcel of public land for a small registration fee. In 1869, the completion of the first transcontinental railroad, connecting the two coasts, marked the true opening of the West. The plains, once attractive only to traders and trappers, were now appealing to farmers, miners, and companies desiring new land. Travelers on trains shot buffalo for sport, and the mighty herds on the prairie diminished rapidly. By 1870, the buffalo were reduced to one-third their original number.

The frontier shrank as settle-

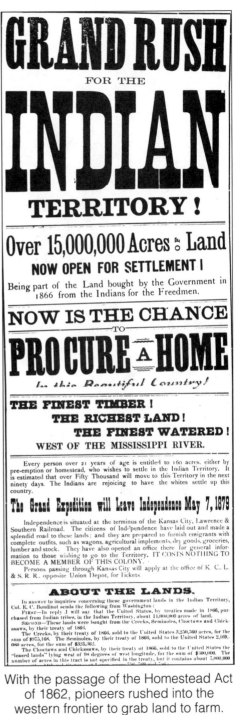

With the passage of the Homestead Act of 1862, pioneers rushed into the western frontier to grab land to farm. In the process, many Indian tribes were displaced.

49

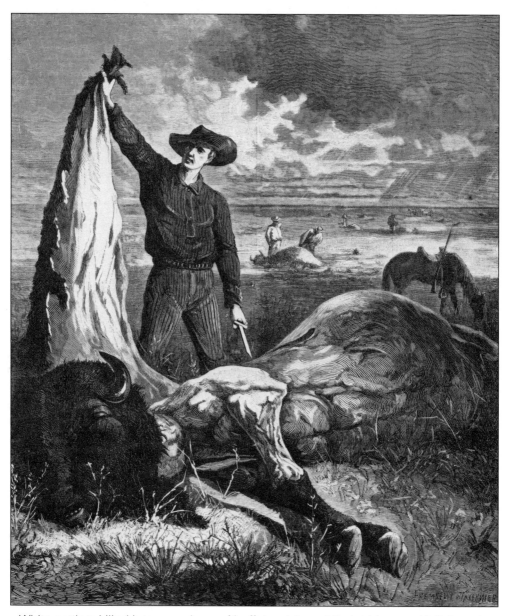

White settlers killed huge numbers of buffalo, stripped their hides, and left them to rot in the sun. To the Indians, this slaughter seemed senseless and immoral.

ments increased. To the white settlers seeking land and opportunity, the Indians were an obstacle to progress. The settlers viewed the Indians as stupid—a people who did not even exploit the bountiful land for farming and business. The army used any excuse to wage war against the tribes, which were weary and confused. They were facing government relocation to new lands, strong competition for food, the introduction of alcohol, and the recurrent smallpox plagues.

In the second half of the century, smallpox epidemics continued to strike the Indians. For example, epidemics in 1869 and 1870 reduced many Indian tribes in Montana, including the Gros Ventres, Blackfoot, and Assiniboin. This time, however, the destruction was not as great as it had been thirty years earlier.

While almost no year passed without some tribe being attacked by the disease, the death rate among Indians from smallpox epidemics eventually began to decrease. One reason for the declining death rate was simply that the survivors of past epidemics became immune to the smallpox virus. Also, fewer Indians suffered from smallpox simply because there were fewer Indians left alive after the previous epidemics.

Another factor that slowed Indian

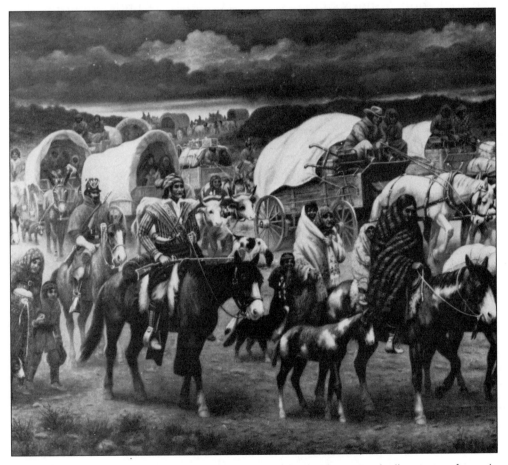

As the frontier shrank under the burgeoning white settlements, Indians were forced to relocate. One of the most infamous of these relocations was the Cherokee Trail of Tears. Many Cherokee Indians died on this march.

deaths was the long-overdue increase in vaccination programs. These programs were administered by government officials known as Indian agents. Indian agents lived in or near villages and reservations and were appointed by the Bureau of Indian Affairs. They were the official contact between tribes and the federal government.

The Indian agents were kept busy during the continuing smallpox plagues. In 1856, an epidemic hit the Kickapoo Indians of Kansas. Twenty-four Indians died. During the epidemic, Indian agents vaccinated the rest of the Kickapoo, saving them from the virus. The few who refused vaccination died. These efforts were repeated with the Yancton Sioux in South Dakota, North Dakota, Wyoming, and Montana in 1859, with the Winnebago Indians of Minnesota in 1860, and with many other tribes throughout the country as the century wore on.

Less Important than Whites

Though vaccination efforts had increased, the government still considered Indians to be less important than whites. In 1880, vaccination became mandatory for white children in Massachusetts and Georgia. But vaccination of Indian children did not become mandatory until after 1907. And in 1882, with more than 300,000 Indians still unvaccinated, the U.S. government spent about fifteen hundred dollars on vaccine. But this amount of money did not buy much vaccine. The following year, an epidemic killed many unvaccinated children at the pueblos of San Ildefonso and San Juan in New Mexico.

By the end of the nineteenth century, though, smallpox was no longer a major problem for the Indians of North America. In fact, after 1900, more unvaccinated whites suffered from smallpox than Indians. Those Indians who had survived earlier plagues were naturally immune to future ones. Those who had not personally suffered from smallpox now understood the danger of infection and accepted vaccination as the one sure way to avoid the deadly disease.

Once Masters of the Land

As the frontier disappeared, the Indians of North America, once masters of the land, now numbered only 350,000, or one-third of 1 percent of the U.S. population.

By the end of the nineteenth century, the United States had become a powerful nation. Many more Europeans arrived, seeing a land full of opportunity. George Catlin saw the masses of new immigrants—the new Americans—and could think only of the first Americans: "Thirty millions of white men are now scuffling for the goods and luxuries of life over the bones and ashes of twelve millions of red men, six millions of whom had fallen victims to the small-pox, and the remainder to the sword, bayonet, or whisky."

According to the 1980 census, 1.5 million Indians live in the United States. Representing a fraction of this number are the descendants of

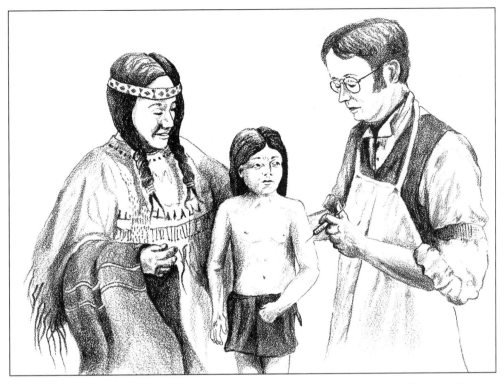

Smallpox gradually became less of a threat to the Indians. In part, this was due to vaccination programs.

the upper Missouri tribes that suffered in the plague from 1837 to 1840. In 1985, the Montana population of Assiniboin numbered about twenty-eight hundred. Their former enemies, the Blackfoot, live on reservations in Montana and Alberta. In 1985, the Montana reservation had a population of about seven thousand. Some Blackfoot live in a reservation in Idaho, too, while more than five thousand live off the reservations.

Epilogue
Future Plagues?

In early 1979, Somalia, East Africa, which had always been plagued by smallpox epidemics, was declared to be free of smallpox. Later that year, the Global Commission for Certification of Smallpox Eradication, formed in 1977 and composed of a panel of medical experts from different countries, stated that smallpox had finally been eradicated all over the world. In 1980, the World Health Assembly, meeting in Geneva, Switzerland, officially supported the momentous announcement. This marked the first time in history that a disease has been removed from the face of the earth by a man-made cure.

Smallpox Could Return

Smallpox, however, might return in a different form. New, fiercer strains of the deadly disease have developed. In fact, a strain limited to West Africa known as monkey pox has been infecting humans since 1970, and scientists are watching it closely.

In addition to new strains of smallpox developing naturally, there are strains that have been developed by scientists for research and study. The writer Joel Shurkin insists that if smallpox returns, it will come from these strains created in laboratories. "There are about eight laboratories in the world with variola viruses locked and frozen for study," said Shurkin. Little glass vials containing virus specimens from many different years and places are stored at ninety-four degrees below zero in guarded vaults. Fearing accidental outbreaks, the World Health Organization has asked several of these laboratories to either destroy their supply of the virus or ship it to a central lab. But for a variety of reasons, the laboratories have refused.

A National Scare

One outbreak of smallpox from a lab has already happened. On February 28, 1973, an Irish laboratory worker named Ann Algeo caught the smallpox virus after being exposed to it at work. She infected several people, one of whom died. The incident triggered a national scare before the disease was under control.

It is clear that germs are easily spread. In a room containing more than one person, everyone in the room takes in, with every breath, dried flakes from the throats of others. Germs also spread to many peo-

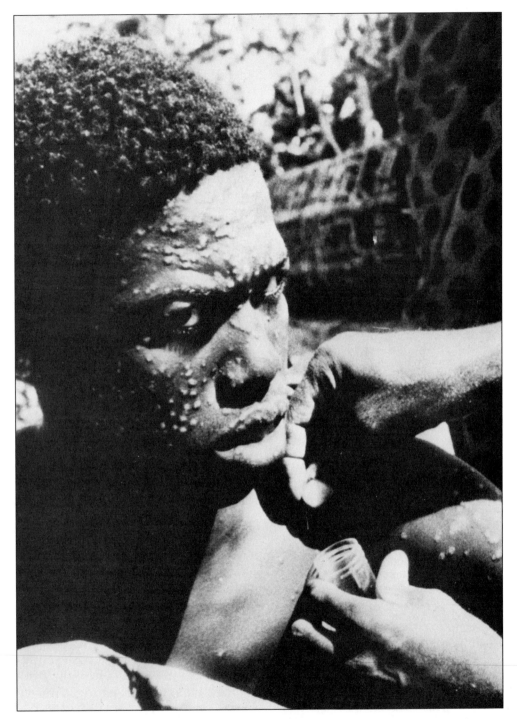

In 1980, the World Health Organization declared smallpox to be eradicated. The last major epidemic occurred in Somalia, East Africa, in 1977.

ple quickly in other enclosed environments, such as subway cars and offices with central air-conditioning systems.

Germs are not only easily spread from person to person but from country to country, too. As people and goods move around the world freely, any major outbreak of a new virus could become a global one. It would not be limited to a certain region, or even a single country. For example, scientists have documented that mosquito larvae from Africa arrived in a jet plane at a Kansas airport. Fortunately the mosquito larvae were not disease-infested. It is thought by some scientists that the devastating AIDS disease was brought to the United States from Haiti, a popular vacation spot among Americans.

What Can We Do?

There are several things people must do to protect themselves from a future smallpox epidemic. First, medical and government authorities must encourage people to continue to be vaccinated. People who live in large industrial nations often do not believe that this and other serious diseases can come back. Governments, too, do not seem concerned with encouraging vaccination. According to Allan Chase, a medical researcher and writer, "More than one-third of this country's over 12 million children under the age of four are deprived each year of available immunizations against polio, diphtheria, tetanus, whooping cough, measles, mumps, and rubella." Children remain unvaccinated for a variety of reasons, including parental ignorance or deep religious beliefs against vaccination.

In early 1991, six children in Philadelphia died of measles. Four of the six were members of the Faith Tabernacle Congregation Church, whose pastor refused to allow the inoculation of his school's two hundred students. The pastor and his

---

REFINEMENTS IN THE VACCINE

Changes have occurred in the smallpox vaccine Edward Jenner developed in 1797. In the 1880s, a British scientist named Monckton Copeman demonstrated that a substance called glycerin could preserve the purity of the vaccine. Until that time, the vaccine often became contaminated by bacteria. But glycerin-protected vaccine had to be kept cool to remain effective. A form of freeze-dried vaccine began to appear in the 1920s. The quality of the vaccine was inconsistent until the process was perfected in 1954.

Attitudes toward the vaccine were slower to change than the vaccine itself. Dr. C.V. Chapin, a Rhode Island epidemiologist—a doctor who studies epidemics and the spread of disease—complained in 1913 that the United States was "the least vaccinated of any civilized country." Public resistance was strong even into the twentieth century. These critics claimed vaccination was worse than the disease because early vaccines often caused people to get the disease.

But in 1922, important legislation began to turn Americans toward the acceptance of vaccination. In that year, the U.S. Supreme Court ruled that school authorities had the right to require vaccination for admission to school at all times, whether there was threat of smallpox or not.

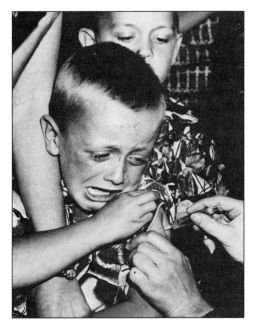

Widespread vaccination has curbed many deadly diseases, including polio, smallpox, and diphtheria.

In Philadelphia, as in most of the United States, children are required to be immunized before going to school, unless their religion prevents it.

Finally, indifference to those already suffering from disease must be overcome. Chase writes that once Edward Jenner discovered smallpox vaccination in 1797, the real reason for the disease's continuance among the Indians was apathy and indifference on the part of whites to the plight of the infected. Many members of the gay community believe a similar indifference exists today. They believe the government will not work as hard to find a cure for AIDS because the disease mostly affects gay men and intravenous drug users, who are shunned by society. If these accusations are right, society may be showing the same type of indifference it showed the Indians during the smallpox epidemic. Only the future can reveal whether people will work together to prevent future epidemics.

congregation do not believe in pursuing medical treatment because it would show distrust in God. Authorities have since closed down the school, and the courts will determine whether a person can indeed be forced to submit to vaccination.

Glossary

cowpox: A contagious disease among cows that produces sores on the udders. A person exposed to cowpox is immune to smallpox.

earth lodge: A dwelling built by the Plains Indians. Circular and partially buried, it was made of logs, tightly bound grasses, and sod. The houses were quite large, and could house several families.

frontier: The region where settled territory meets the wilderness.

hemorrhagic smallpox: The most severe form of smallpox, usually resulting in death. The smallpox pustules attack the internal organs, causing hemorrhage.

Homestead Act: Enacted in 1862, the act allowed U.S. citizens to gain free title to land they had lived on and cultivated for five years. Indians could also gain land under the Homestead Act, but only if they completely renounced their tribal connections.

immunity: The body's ability to resist disease. To achieve immunity to the smallpox virus, vaccinia is injected into the body, which stimulates the body's immune system. The immune system then produces antibodies to the virus. These antibodies remain in the system to fight any future attack of the virus.

Indian Removal Act: Enacted by the administration of President Andrew Jackson in 1830, the act allowed for the forced removal of all Indians east of the Mississippi River to newly created Indian territory west of the river. (Indian territory was composed of present-day Arkansas and Oklahoma.)

inoculation: Practice used for centuries to protect a person from catching a disease. The process involves injecting a healthy person with a mild form of the disease in order to build up the body's resistance.

pustule: A slight, inflamed elevation of the skin filled with pus. In the worst cases of smallpox, pustules covered a victim's entire body.

smallpox: A highly contagious disease characterized by high fever, severe rash, and sores which leave scars.

sweat baths: A religious or healing ritual that took place in a sweat lodge, a small round structure of sticks or hide. Inside the lodge, water was poured over fire-heated rocks, producing steam which was meant to purify the body. After being exposed to the steam, an individual plunged into snow or a cold stream.

tepee: A cone-shaped tent constructed from animal hides and used as living quarters by the Plains Indians.

vaccine: Preparation of either live or dead virus, bacteria, or other chemicals that increases the body's immunity to a particular disease.

vaccinia: Virus used in smallpox vaccination. Vaccinia mutated from the cowpox virus sometime in the last two hundred years. It is also the largest virus known to man—it can be seen without an electron microscope.

variola virus: Variola (Latin for "spotted") is the name for the three main smallpox-causing viruses: variola major, variola intermedia, and variola minor.

virus: A tiny organism capable of entering and destroying healthy living cells. By using the material of a healthy cell, a virus is able to reproduce and spread throughout the body, causing disease.

Suggestions for Further Reading

Chittenden, H. M., *History of Early Steamboat Navigation on the Missouri River; Life and Adventures of Joseph La Barge, Vol. 1*. New York: F. P. Harper, 1903.

Ewers, John, *The Blackfeet: Raiders on the Northwestern Plains*. Norman: University of Oklahoma Press, 1958.

Larpenteur, Charles, *Forty Years a Fur Trader on the Upper Missouri*. Lincoln: University of Nebraska Press, 1989.

White, Jon Manchip, *Everyday Life of the North American Indian*. New York: Holmes & Meier, 1979.

Wilson, Elinor, *Jim Beckwourth: Black Mountain Man and War Chief of the Crows*. Norman: University of Oklahoma Press, 1972.

Wissler, Clark, *Indians of the United States*. New York: Doubleday, 1966.

Works Consulted

Athearn, Robert G., *Forts of the Upper Missouri*. Englewood Cliffs, NJ: Prentice-Hall, 1967.

Catlin, George, *North American Indians*. New York: Viking-Penguin, 1989.

Chardon, F. A., *Journal at Fort Clark, 1834-1839*. Edited by Annie H. Abel. Pierre: South Dakota State Department of History, 1932.

Chase, Allan, *Magic Shots*. New York: William Morrow, 1982.

Dateline: CDC, Vol. 11, No. 10. Atlanta: Centers for Disease Control, October 1979.

DeVoto, Bernard, *Across the Wide Missouri*. Boston: Houghton Mifflin, 1947.

Hopkins, Donald, *Princes and Peasants*. Chicago: University of Chicago Press, 1983.

Kennedy, Dan, *Recollections of an Assiniboine Chief*. Toronto: McClelland & Stewart, 1972.

Lamar, Howard, and Leonard Thompson, eds. *The Frontier in History*. New Haven, CT: Yale University Press, 1981.

Meyer, Roy H., *The Village Indians of the Upper Missouri*. Lincoln: University of Nebraska Press, 1977.

Shurkin, Joel N., *The Invisible Fire*. New York: G. P. Putnam's Sons, 1979.

Thomas, Dave, and Karin Ronnefeldt, eds. *People of the First Man: Life Among the Plains Indians in Their Final Days of Glory*. New York: E. P. Dutton, 1976.

Index

About the Author

Arthur Diamond, born in Queens, New York, has lived and worked in Colorado, New Mexico, and Oregon. He received a bachelor's degree in English from the University of Oregon and a master's degree in English/Writing from Queens College. A former book editor in New York City, Mr. Diamond is the author of several nonfiction books, including another published by Lucent Books, *The Bhopal Chemical Leak*. A writer and teacher in Queens, he currently lives in his boyhood home with his wife, Irina, and their children, Benjamin Thomas, and Jessica Ann.

Picture Credits